"Nurturing Love: A Stay-Married Devotional for Couples"

I0408512

Nadia Ari

Table of Contents:

Chapter 1: Planting Seeds of Love: Cultivating a Foundation for Lasting Marriage

Introduction:

A successful and continuing marriage is erected upon a strong foundation of love, trust, and commitment. Just as a gardener nurtures a seed to grow into a beautiful factory, couples must also invest time and trouble in cultivating their relationship. This chapter explores the essential rudiments of planting seeds of love in a marriage, furnishing practical perceptivity and guidance for couples seeking to make a solid foundation that withstands the tests of time.

Understanding the significance of a Foundation
A foundation is the bedrock on which a structure stands, furnishing stability and support. also, a solid foundation is pivotal

for a lasting marriage. This section delves into the significance of a strong foundation, emphasizing the part it plays in fostering a healthy and thriving relationship.

Cultivating Communication
Effective communication is the lifeblood of any successful marriage. Couples must learn to express their studies, passions, and needs openly and actually. This section explores colorful communication ways, similar as active listening,non-verbal cues, and formative dialogue, to help couples foster healthy and meaningful communication.

Building Trust Brick by Brick
Trust forms the foundation of a lasting marriage. Without trust, a relationship becomes vulnerable and fragile. This section delves into the significance of trust- structure exercises, fostering translucency, and demonstrating trustability to establish a strong sense of trust within the marriage.

Nurturing Emotional Connection
Emotional closeness is the cement that holds a marriage together. Couples must

prioritize nurturing their emotional connection, fostering empathy, and understanding each other's emotional requirements. This section offers practical suggestions for creating emotional closeness through quality time, participated gests , and emotional vulnerability.

Strengthening the Bond through Shared Values
Shared values give a common frame and sense of purpose for couples. This section explores the significance of aligning values and discusses styles to identify and cultivate participated values within a marriage, allowing couples to grow together in harmony.

Cultivating Friendship and Partnership
Friendship serves as a foundation for a strong and continuing marriage. This section highlights the significance of cultivating fellowship, enjoying participated pursuits and interests, and supporting each other's growth. It also addresses the need for balance between individuality and togetherness in a marriage.

Navigating Conflict and Resolving Differences
Conflict is ineluctable in any relationship, but how couples handle it determines the strength of their foundation. This section delves into effective conflict resolution strategies, emphasizing the significance of regardful communication, concession, and remission.

Fostering closeness and love
closeness and love are essential aspects of a thriving marriage. This section explores the significance of physical and emotional closeness, offering practical tips to reignite passion and keep the honey of love alive.

Investing in Self- Growth and Personal Development
Individual growth contributes to the growth of a marriage. This section emphasizes the significance of tone-mindfulness, tone- care, and particular development within the environment of a relationship. It provides perceptivity on how couples can support each other's growth and produce an terrain conducive to individual fulfillment.

Cultivating Gratitude and Appreciation
Gratitude and appreciation act as toxin
for a lasting marriage. This section
highlights the power of expressing
gratefulness, admitting each other's
sweats, and cultivating a culture of
appreciation within the relationship.

Chapter 2: Watering the Garden: Communication as Nourishment for Love

Introduction:

Effective communication serves as the lifeblood of a healthy and thriving relationship. Just as water nourishes a theater , communication nourishes love and connection within a marriage. This chapter explores the significance of communication as a vital element of a successful relationship. It delves into colorful aspects of communication, furnishing practical perceptivity and guidance for couples to enhance their communication chops and consolidate their bond of love.

The Power of Open and Honest Communication
Open and honest communication forms the foundation of a strong and nurturing relationship. This section emphasizes the significance of creating a safe andnon-

judgmental space for expressing studies, passions, and needs. It explores the benefits of transparent communication and the mischievous goods of withholding or miscommunicating.

Active harkening The crucial to Understanding
Active listening is a abecedarian skill that enhances communication and fosters understanding between mates. This section delves into the art of active listening, pressing the significance of giving concentrated attention, rehearsing empathy, and seeking explanation. It provides practical tips for couples to develop active listening chops and demonstrate genuine interest in each other's perspectives.

Non-Verbal Communication The Unspoken Language of Love
Non-verbal cues play a significant part in conveying feelings, intentions, and solicitations. This section explores the nuances ofnon-verbal communication, including body language, facial expressions, and gestures. It emphasizes the need to be aware ofnon-verbal cues and encourages couples to develop

mindfulness and understanding of each other'snon-verbal communication.

Effective Expression of passions and Needs

Expressing passions and requirements in a clear and formative manner is essential for maintaining emotional closeness in a relationship. This section provides practical strategies for couples to articulate their feelings effectively, avoid blame or review, and express requirements without creating guard or resentment. It emphasizes the power of" I" statements and encourages couples to validate and admire each other's feelings.

The Art of Conflict Resolution

Conflict is an ineluctable part of any relationship, but how couples handle conflicts determines the strength and life of their love. This section explores effective conflict resolution ways, similar as active listening, concession, and chancing palm- palm results. It emphasizes the significance of maintaining respect, empathy, and understanding during dissensions , and offers guidance onde-escalating conflicts and chancing common ground.

Honesty and Trust Building Blocks of Communication
Honesty and trust are intertwined with effective communication. This section explores the part of honesty in fostering trust and heightening the connection between mates. It highlights the significance of being veracious, responsible, and dependable in communication and addresses the challenges of rebuilding trust after breaches or backstabbings.

aware Communication Being Present in the Moment
awareness plays a pivotal part in enhancing communication. This section delves into the practice of aware communication, emphasizing the significance of being completely present, attentive, andnon-judgmental during exchanges. It provides practical exercises and ways for couples to cultivate awareness in their communication, leading to deeper understanding and connection.

Communicating Love and Appreciation

Communication isn't only about addressing conflicts or agitating serious matters; it's also a tool for expressing love, affection, and appreciation. This section explores the significance of verbal andnon-verbal expressions of love and offers suggestions for couples to incorporate diurnal acts of appreciation and gratefulness into their communication.

prostrating Communication walls Communication walls can hamper the inflow of understanding and love between mates. This section identifies common communication walls, similar as guard, unresistant- aggressiveness, and lack of fierceness. It provides strategies for prostrating these walls, including active tone- reflection, seeking professional help if demanded, and nurturing tolerance and empathy.

Cultivating Emotional closeness through Communication
Emotional closeness is nurtured through deep and meaningful communication. This section explores the link between emotional closeness and effective communication, emphasizing the

significance of vulnerability, empathy, and active engagement in exchanges. It provides guidance for couples to produce a safe space for participating feelings, dreams, and fears, thereby fostering a deeper emotional connection.

Chapter 3: Tending to the Soil: Prioritizing Emotional Connection

Introduction:

In a healthy and fulfilling relationship, emotional connection acts as the soil that nurtures love, closeness, and understanding. Just as a gardener tends to the soil to insure the growth of vibrant and healthy shops, couples must prioritize the civilization of emotional connection in their relationship. This chapter explores the significance of emotional connection and provides practical perceptivity and guidance for couples to prioritize and nurture this essential aspect of their cooperation.

Understanding Emotional Connection Emotional connection refers to the deep bond and sense of understanding that exists between mates. This section explores the significance of emotional connection in fostering trust, closeness, and overall relationship satisfaction. It highlights the part of emotional connection in promoting empathy, support, and collective growth within a relationship.

Cultivating Emotional mindfulness
Developing emotional mindfulness is pivotal for fostering emotional connection. This section delves into the process of tone- reflection and soul-searching, helping individualities identify and understand their own feelings. It also explores the significance of being attuned to and open to the feelings of one's mate, fostering empathy and deeper understanding.

Open and Vulnerable Communication
Open and vulnerable communication serves as a catalyst for erecting emotional connection. This section emphasizes the significance of creating a safe andnon-judgmental space for participating studies, fears, dreams, and vulnerabilities. It explores the power of active listening, validating feelings, and offering support, thereby heightening the emotional bond between mates.

Quality Time and Shared gests

Spending quality time together and engaging in participated gests strengthens emotional connection. This section explores the significance of sculpturing out devoted time for each other, down from distractions and diurnal liabilities. It highlights the value of engaging in conditioning that foster connection and produce lasting recollections, similar as date nights, participated pursuits, and exploring new adventures together.

Expressing Appreciation and Gratitude
Expressing appreciation and gratefulness nourishes emotional connection within a relationship. This section delves into the power of admitting and appreciating each other's sweats, strengths, and benefactions. It provides guidance on incorporating gratefulness practices into diurnal life, fostering a positive and appreciative atmosphere that strengthens the emotional bond between mates.

Nurturing Emotional Support
furnishing emotional support is essential for cultivating emotional connection. This section explores the significance of being there for each other during both joyous

and grueling times. It discusses the significance of active empathy, validating feelings, and offering comfort and consolation, thereby fostering a sense of security and trust within the relationship.

Creating Rituals of Connection
Rituals of connection serve as anchors for emotional connection within a relationship. This section highlights the value of creating participated rituals, similar as diurnal check- sways, daily reflection sessions, or special traditions, to consolidate emotional closeness. It provides practical suggestions for incorporating rituals of connection into diurnal life, icing harmonious aliment of the emotional bond.

Fostering Trust and Intimacy
Trust and closeness are nearly intertwined with emotional connection. This section explores the significance of trust- structure exercises, cultivating translucency, and nurturing physical and emotional closeness. It emphasizes the part of vulnerability, respect, and heightening emotional connection as foundations for erecting trust and

fostering closeness within the relationship.

Supporting Each Other's Growth
Emotional connection supports and encourages particular growth within a cooperation. This section delves into the significance of nurturing individual bournes and pretensions while remaining connected as a couple. It highlights the part of emotional support, stimulant, and active engagement in each other's particular development, fostering a sense of collective growth and fulfillment.

prostrating Challenges to Emotional Connection
Challenges can arise that hamper emotional connection in a relationship. This section addresses common obstacles, similar as conflicts, stress, and external pressures, and provides guidance on navigating and prostrating them. It emphasizes the significance of open communication, empathy, and adaptability in maintaining and strengthening emotional connection during delicate times.

Chapter 4: Sowing Trust: Building a Solid Ground for Intimacy

Introduction:

Trust forms the bedrock of a healthy and intimate relationship. It acts as the foundation upon which emotional closeness and vulnerability thrive. Just as a planter sows seeds to cultivate a bountiful crop, couples must sow trust to make a solid ground for closeness. This chapter explores the significance of trust in fostering closeness and provides practical perceptivity and guidance for couples to strengthen and cultivate trust within their relationship.

Understanding the significance of Trust Trust serves as the foundation of a successful and fulfilling relationship. This section delves into the significance of trust, emphasizing its part in fostering emotional safety, vulnerability, and overall relationship satisfaction. It explores how trust enhances communication, deepens emotional connection, and promotes collective growth and support.

thickness and trustability
thickness and trustability are crucial factors of erecting trust. This section discusses the significance of following through on commitments, being reliable, and demonstrating harmonious geste
. It highlights the value of maintaining integrity and trustability in conduct and words, therefore establishing a solid foundation of trust.

Open and Honest Communication
Open and honest communication is essential for erecting trust within a relationship. This section explores the significance of transparent and veracious dialogue. It discusses the significance of creating a safe andnon-judgmental space for open communication, where both mates feel comfortable expressing their studies, passions, and enterprises.

Trust- Building Exercises
Trust can be designedly nurtured through colorful exercises and conditioning. This section provides practical suggestions for

trust- structure exercises, similar as rehearsing active listening, participating vulnerabilities, and engaging in trust-structure games or exercises. It emphasizes the part of these conditioning in fostering understanding, empathy, and collective trust between mates.

Building Trust through Emotional Support
furnishing emotional support is pivotal for erecting trust within a relationship. This section explores the significance of laboriously harkening, offering empathy, and furnishing a safe space for each other's feelings. It highlights the part of emotional support in strengthening the emotional bond and cultivating trust.

Honesty and translucency
Honesty and translucency are vital constituents in structure and maintaining trust. This section delves into the significance of being honest with one another, indeed in delicate situations. It discusses the value of translucency, participating information openly, and avoiding dishonesty or hidden dockets, which contribute to the development of trust within the relationship.

Trust- Building After Betrayal
Rebuilding trust after a breach or treason can be a grueling process. This section provides guidance for couples navigating trust restoration. It discusses the significance of responsibility, remission, and harmonious trouble in rebuilding trust. It emphasizes the need for open communication, tolerance, and understanding during this mending trip.

Trust and Boundaries
Establishing and esteeming boundaries is nearly tied to erecting trust. This section explores the relationship between trust and boundaries, emphasizing the significance of establishing clear prospects, recognizing particular boundaries, and maintaining respect for each other's requirements and limits.

Demonstrating responsibility responsibility is the incarnation of trust in action. This section discusses the actions and rates that contribute to being seen as secure by one's mate. It explores the significance of trustability, honesty, fidelity, and thickness as trust- structure attributes.

Nurturing Trust through Shared
Experiences
Shared gests play a part in structure and
buttressing trust within a relationship.
This section explores the significance of
creating positive recollections, engaging
in participated conditioning, and fostering
a sense of cooperation and cooperation. It
emphasizes the part of participated gests
in strengthening the emotional bond and
cultivating trust.

Chapter 5: Pruning and Grafting: Overcoming Challenges Together

Introduction:

Challenges are an ineluctable part of any relationship. Just as a gardener prunes and grafts shops to insure their growth and health, couples must also face challenges head- on and work together to overcome them. This chapter explores the significance of facing challenges as a platoon and provides practical perceptivity and guidance for couples on how to navigate obstacles and strengthen their bond through the process.

Embracing Challenges as Growth openings
Challenges, although delicate, give openings for particular and relational growth. This section discusses the significance of reframing challenges as openings for literacy, adaptability, and strengthening the relationship. It emphasizes the mindset shift demanded

to view challenges as stepping monuments to a deeper connection.

Effective Communication During Challenges
Clear and effective communication is pivotal when facing challenges as a couple. This section explores the significance of open and honest communication during delicate times. It provides practical strategies for active listening, expressing feelings constructively, and working together to find results.

Developing Adaptability and Rigidity
Adaptability and rigidity are crucial rates for prostrating challenges together. This section discusses the significance of developing adaptability as a couple and chancing the strength to bounce back from lapses. It explores strategies for erecting adaptability, similar as maintaining a positive outlook, seeking support, and conforming to changing circumstances.

Cultivating Empathy and Understanding
Empathy and understanding are essential when facing challenges as a platoon. This

section delves into the significance of putting oneself in the shoes of the mate, seeking to understand their perspective, and offering support and confirmation. It explores strategies for cultivating empathy, fostering compassion, and heightening understanding.

cooperative Problem- working cooperative problem- solving is a important tool for prostrating challenges together. This section discusses the benefits of working as a platoon to find results and make common opinions. It explores ways similar as brainstorming, compromising, and seeking palm- palm issues to attack challenges effectively.

Seeking Professional Help
Some challenges may bear professional guidance and support. This section emphasizes the significance of feting when outside help is demanded and seeking the backing of therapists or counselors. It discusses the part of professional support in furnishing tools, perceptivity, and guidance to navigate challenges in a healthy and productive manner.

Fostering Trust and Unity
Trust and concinnity are vital when facing
challenges as a couple. This section
explores strategies for structure and
maintaining trust during delicate times. It
emphasizes the significance of
demonstrating trustability, honesty, and
responsibility to strengthen the
foundation of trust. It also highlights the
significance of staying united as a platoon,
facing challenges together rather than
turning against each other.

tone- Care and collective Support
tone- care and collective support are
essential for adaptability and well- being
when prostrating challenges. This section
explores the significance of tone- care
practices, similar as managing stress,
maintaining particular interests, and
seeking support outside the relationship.
It emphasizes the part of furnishing
collective support and being each other's
source of strength during grueling times.

literacy and Growing Together
Challenges can come openings for growth
and literacy as a couple. This section
discusses the significance of reflecting on
challenges, relating assignments learned,

and applying them to unborn situations. It encourages couples to view challenges as a participated trip of growth and discovery, strengthening their bond along the way.

Celebrating Successes and mileposts Celebrating successes and mileposts is pivotal to admit progress and foster positivity during grueling times. This section explores the significance of feting and celebrating achievements, both big and small. It emphasizes the significance of expressing gratefulness, admitting sweats, and reflecting on the couple's adaptability and growth throughout the challenges faced.

Chapter 6: Fertilizing Friendship: Growing Strong Companionship

Introduction:

Fellowship is a cherished bond that enriches our lives, furnishing support, horselaugh, and a sense of belonging. Like a delicate factory, a fellowship requires nurturing, care, and regular feeding to grow strong and flourish. This composition explores the colorful aspects of cultivating and fertilizing fellowship to establish and maintain robust camaraderie.

I. The Seed of fellowship

Chancing Common Ground
Friendship frequently begins with participated interests, pursuits, or values. relating common ground helps make a foundation on which a fellowship can thrive. Engaging in conditioning together, similar as sports, music, or volunteering,

facilitates cling and establishes a sense of belonging.

Authenticity and Trust
Authenticity forms the bedrock of fellowship. Being genuine and honest in relations fosters trust. Trust is a pivotal element that strengthens fellowship, allowing individualities to calculate on each other and entrust in one another without fear of judgment.

II. soddening the Roots Communication and Emotional Support

Open and Honest Communication
Effective communication is vital in any relationship. musketeers must be suitable to express their studies, passions, and enterprises openly. laboriously harkening and offering support and understanding helps musketeers feel valued and strengthens their connection.

Emotional Support
gemütlichkeit flourish when individualities give emotional support during grueling times. Offering a sympathetic observance, showing empathy, and furnishing consolation

cultivates a sense of security within the fellowship.

III. Cultivating Growth Quality Time and Shared gests

Quality Time
Spending quality time together is a foundation of fellowship. Engaging in conditioning that both musketeers enjoy, similar as going for walks, exploring new places, or simply having meaningful exchanges, nurtures the bond and deepens the connection.

Shared gests
participating gests , both positive and negative, creates lasting recollections and strengthens the fellowship. Celebrating mileposts, prostrating obstacles together, and creating new adventures cultivates a sense of fellowship and participated history.

IV. Weeding Out Negativity Resolving Conflicts

Conflict Resolution
Conflicts are ineluctable in any relationship, but addressing them

instantly and hypercritically is pivotal. musketeers must learn to communicate their enterprises, hear to each other's perspectives, and work towards chancing mutually agreeable results. Resolving conflicts strengthens the fellowship by fostering understanding and growth.

Letting Go of poisonous connections occasionally, despite our sweats, gemütlichkeit can turn poisonous. Feting the signs of poisonous geste , similar as manipulation, discourteousness, or constant negativity, is essential. In similar cases, prioritizing one's well- being and letting go of poisonous gemütlichkeit is necessary for particular growth and fostering healthier connections.

Fertilizing the Soil Support and festivity

Support and stimulant
Being there for musketeers in times of need is pivotal to maintaining a healthy fellowship. Supporting each other's pretensions, dreams, and bournes helps foster a nurturing terrain where both individualities can thrive.

Celebrating mileposts
Celebrating each other's accomplishments, big or small, is an important aspect of fellowship. Feting achievements and participating in the joy reinforces the bond and fosters a culture of positivity and stimulant.

VI. raying Out Expanding the Circle

Encouraging Addition
Expanding the fellowship circle to include new individualities is a sign of maturity and openness. Encouraging inclusivity within the group strengthens the bond by diversifying perspectives and introducing new gests .

Cultivating Individual gemütlichkeit
While group gemütlichkeit are precious, it's essential to foster individual connections within the group. Spending one- on- one time with musketeers helps consolidate the understanding of each other's unique rates, strengthening the overall fellowship.

Chapter 7: Basking in the Sun: Celebrating Joy and Laughter in Marriage

Introduction:

Marriage is a beautiful trip filled with love, fellowship, and participated gests . While it may have its fair share of challenges, celebrating joy and horselaugh is essential to maintaining a strong and fulfilling connubial bond. In this composition, we claw into the significance of humor, naturalness, and chancing joy in marriage. We explore how horselaugh can bring couples closer, enhance their emotional connection, and produce a flexible foundation for a lasting and joyful union.

I. The Power of horselaugh in Marriage

Strengthening Emotional Connection horselaugh acts as a important cement, fostering emotional closeness between mates. participating moments of joy and recreation helps couples bond on a deeper position, erecting a strong foundation of trust, understanding, and participated happiness.

Reducing Stress and Pressure horselaugh serves as a natural stress-reliever, diffusing pressure and promoting a positive atmosphere within the marriage. In moments of stress, humor can serve as a managing medium, allowing couples to navigate grueling situations with a lighter heart and a more auspicious outlook.

II. Embracing Humor in Everyday Life

prankishness and naturalness Cultivating a sense of prankishness and naturalness in everyday life injects joy into the marriage. Engaging in silly capers, participating sportful badinage, or surprising each other with unconcerned gestures keeps the relationship vibrant and helps break down from the humdrum of diurnal routines.

Chancing Humor in the Mundane

Mundane conditioning can be converted into sources of horselaugh and enjoyment. From cooking together and making funny mishaps in the kitchen to chancing humor in ménage chores, couples can inoculate humor into their everyday tasks, making them more pleasurable and fostering a sense of participated recreation.

III. Shared Adventures and Making Memories

Exploring New gests
Going on adventures together creates openings for participated horselaugh and joy. Whether it's traveling to new destinations, trying new conditioning, or embarking on robotic jaunts, the exhilaration of new gests frequently leads to participated horselaugh and memorable moments that strengthen the connubial bond.

Creating Traditions and Rituals
Establishing unique traditions and rituals within the marriage cultivates a sense of joy and expectation. Whether it's a yearly game night, a monthly holiday

, or a quirky anniversary festivity, these rituals give a platform for couples to lounge in participated horselaugh, creating continuing recollections along the way.

IV. Communication and Humor

Wit and badinage
Engaging in light- hearted badinage and sportful teasing can add a touch of humor to everyday exchanges. Quick wit and inoffensive jokes produce a positive and pleasurable atmosphere, allowing couples to communicate with ease and enjoy each other's company.

Humor as a Conflict Resolution Tool
Humor can be a precious tool in diffusing conflicts and defusing tense situations. The capability to fit humor into dissensions helps couples take a step back, gain perspective, and find common ground. Shared horselaugh can pave the way for open communication, leading to effective conflict resolution.

horselaugh as a Form of tone- Care

Stress Relief and Health Benefits

horselaugh has multitudinous health benefits, including stress reduction, increased endorphin release, and bettered cardiovascular health. By participating horselaugh with their partner, couples not only enhance their well- being but also strengthen their relationship.

Boosting Adaptability
A marriage that embraces horselaugh and joy is more flexible in the face of challenges. The capability to find humor during tough times helps couples maintain a positive outlook, bounce back from lapses, and support each other through delicate situations.

VI. Sustaining the Joy Nurturing the horselaugh

Prioritizing Quality Time
Setting away devoted quality time for each other allows couples to reconnect, laugh, and enjoy participated conditioning. Date nights, weekend lams, or indeed cozy nights at home give openings for couples to sustain the joy and horselaugh in their marriage.

Embracing Individual Humor
Feting and appreciating each other's
unique sense of humor is vital.
Understanding what makes your mate
laugh and laboriously engaging in
conditioning that bring them joy
strengthens the bond and keeps the
horselaugh alive.

Chapter 8: Navigating Storms: Weathering Trials and Tough Times

Introduction:

Life is a trip that encompasses both smooth sailing and turbulent storms. Trials and tough times are ineluctable, and how we navigate through them determines our adaptability and growth. In this composition, we claw into the significance of riding storms, exploring strategies and stations that help us navigate challenges and crop stronger on the other side. From cultivating adaptability and seeking support to rehearsing tone- care and maintaining a positive mindset, we uncover the tools necessary for successfully navigating life's storms.

Understanding the Nature of Storms

Acceptance of evanescence

Storms, whether they be particular, professional, or particular, are part of the mortal experience. Accepting that challenges will arise and change is ineluctable allows us to approach them with a more balanced mindset.

Feting Growth openings
Trials and tough times give openings for particular growth and tone- discovery. By embracing challenges as chances to learn, acclimatize, and develop adaptability, we can find meaning and purpose indeed in the midst of delicate situations.

II. Cultivating Adaptability

structure Emotional Strength
Adaptability is the capability to bounce back from adversity. Strengthening emotional adaptability involves cultivating a positive mindset, rehearsing tone- compassion, and developing effective managing mechanisms similar as awareness, journaling, or seeking remedy when demanded.

Embracing Change and Rigidity
The capability to acclimatize to new circumstances and embrace change is

pivotal during grueling times. flexible individualities are flexible, open- inclined, and willing to acclimate their perspectives and approaches as demanded.

III. Seeking Support Systems

Cultivating Healthy connections structure and maintaining a network of probative connections is essential for riding storms. musketeers, family members, instructors, or support groups can give emotional support, practical advice, and a sense of belonging during tough times.

Professional Support
Seeking professional help, similar as remedy or comforting, can offer precious guidance and backing during grueling ages. Mental health professionals are equipped with the tools and moxie to help individualities navigate delicate feelings and give managing strategies acclimatized to their specific requirements.

IV. rehearsing tone- Care

Prioritizing Physical Well- being

Taking care of our physical health is essential during tough times. Engaging in regular exercise, maintaining a balanced diet, getting enough sleep, and managing stress through relaxation ways can ameliorate adaptability and give the energy demanded to navigate challenges effectively.

Nurturing Emotional Well- being
Emotional tone- care involves rehearsing tone- compassion, setting boundaries, and engaging in conditioning that bring joy and relaxation. This may include pursuits, creative outlets, spending time in nature, or rehearsing awareness and contemplation.

Developing managing Strategies

Problem- working Chops
Developing effective problem- working chops allows individualities to approach challenges in a structured and logical manner. Breaking down problems into manageable way, seeking advice when demanded, and considering different perspectives can grease the process of chancing results.

Embracing a Positive Mindset
Maintaining a positive outlook and
reframing challenges as openings for
growth can significantly impact how we
ride storms. espousing an auspicious
mindset helps cultivate adaptability,
encourages creative problem- working,
and reduces the impact of negative
feelings.

VI. Chancing Meaning and Purpose

Reflecting on particular Values
During tough times, reflecting on our
particular values and aligning our
conduct with them can give a sense of
direction and purpose. Clarifying what
truly matters to us allows us to make
choices that are in line with our core
beliefs, furnishing a sense of meaning
indeed amidst adversity.

Cultivating Gratitude
rehearsing gratefulness shifts our focus
from what's lacking to what we have. By
admitting the positive aspects of our lives,
indeed during delicate times, we can
cultivate adaptability and find moments
of joy, fostering a sense of stopgap and
well- being.

VII. Learning from the Storms

tone- Reflection and Growth
After riding a storm, taking time to reflect on the experience can give precious perceptivity and assignments. Admitting particular growth, relating strengths and areas for enhancement, and setting new pretensions can pave the way for unborn adaptability and success.

participating and Inspiring Others participating our stories and gests can inspire and offer support to others facing analogous challenges. By offering a helping hand, furnishing guidance, or simply being a harkening observance, we can contribute to the collaborative strength and adaptability of our communities.

Chapter 9: Cultivating Forgiveness: Healing Wounds and Restoring Love

Introduction:

Remission is a profound act of mending and restoration that holds the power to mend broken connections, heal emotional injuries, and promote particular growth. In this composition, we claw into the transformative nature of remission, exploring the significance of cultivating remission in our lives. We examine the benefits of remission, the process of forgiving oneself and others, and the profound impact it has on connections and overall well- being. By embracing remission, we can embark on a trip of mending, restoration, and the renewal of love.

Understanding remission

Defining remission

remission is the conscious decision to release passions of resentment, wrathfulness, and the desire for vengeance towards those who have caused us detriment. It involves letting go of negative feelings and choosing to replace them with empathy, understanding, and compassion.

Distinguishing remission from Reconciliation

Forgiveness is distinct from conciliation, which involves restoring a relationship to its former state. remission can do singly, without the necessity of reestablishing the relationship. It's a particular process that allows for mending and growth, anyhow of the outgrowth of the relationship.

II. The Benefits of remission

Emotional Healing and Liberation

Forgiveness liberates us from the burden of carrying resentment, wrathfulness, and bitterness. By releasing these negative feelings, we produce space for emotional mending, inner peace, and particular growth.

bettered Mental Health
Engaging in remission appreciatively impacts internal well- being. It reduces stress, anxiety, and depression, leading to bettered overall cerebral health and increased life satisfaction.

III. The Process of Forgiving

Admitting the Hurt
The first step towards remission is admitting the pain caused by the offense. Validating our feelings and feting the impact of the wrongdoing allows us to defy the hurt and initiate the mending process.

Empathy and Perspective- Taking
Cultivating empathy and trying to understand the perspective of the person who caused the detriment is pivotal. This compassionate approach enables us to humanize the lawbreaker and develop a broader understanding of the circumstances girding the hurtful conduct.

IV. Forgiving Oneself

Self- Compassion

Self- remission is a vital aspect of mending. Cultivating tone- compassion involves treating ourselves with kindness and understanding, admitting our defects, and offering remission for our own miscalculations and failings.

literacy and Growth
Forgiving oneself allows for particular growth and tone- enhancement. It involves feting once miscalculations, taking responsibility for one's conduct, and committing to learning from those gests to make positive changes moving forward.

Forgiving Others

Letting Go of Resentment
Releasing resentment towards those who have harmed us is essential for the remission process. This involves purposely choosing to let go of negative feelings, freeing ourselves from the emotional weight associated with the offense.

Communication and Reconciliation(Optional)

still, remission can lead to conciliation, If the relationship is meaningful and both parties are willing. Open and honest communication, expressing one's passions, and establishing boundaries are essential way in rebuilding trust and restoring the relationship.

VI. The part of Empathy and Compassion

Cultivating Empathy
Empathy plays a pivotal part in the remission process. By putting ourselves in the shoes of the person who caused detriment, we can develop a deeper understanding of their provocations, circumstances, and struggles. This understanding helps foster compassion and facilitates the remission trip.

Compassion towards Others and Ourselves
Compassion is an essential element of remission. Extending compassion to both the lawbreaker and ourselves allows for mending and promotes a sense of interconnectedness and understanding.

VII. Maintaining remission

Accepting fault
Feting that remission is an ongoing
process is vital. It requires acceptance
that lapses and moments ofre-triggering
may do. Embracing fault and allowing
ourselves to continue the mending trip
with tolerance and tone- compassion is
essential.

Setting Boundaries
remission doesn't mean immolating
particular boundaries or subjugating
oneself to repeated detriment. Setting
clear and healthy boundaries is necessary
to maintain tone- respect and cover one's
well- being.

VIII. The Transformative Power of
Forgiveness in connections

Rebuilding Trust
Forgiveness can lay the foundation for
rebuilding trust in connections. It offers
an occasion for the lawbreaker to
demonstrate growth, guilt, and a
commitment to change, thereby fostering
a more flexible and secure connection.

Strengthening Emotional closeness

Through remission, couples can consolidate their emotional bond by participating vulnerabilities, fostering open communication, and supporting each other's particular growth. The process can lead to a lesser sense of emotional closeness and understanding.

IX. Extending remission in a Broader environment

Social and Community Healing Forgiveness extends beyond individual connections and can have a significant impact on societal mending. By promoting remission and empathy in the larger community, we contribute to a more harmonious and compassionate society.

Global Reconciliation
The power of remission has been demonstrated in multitudinous literal exemplifications of conciliation, promoting peace and mending in societies deeply affected by conflict or injustice. remission serves as a catalyst for collaborative mending and the forestallment of cycles of violence.

Chapter 10: Harvesting Gratitude: Cultivating Appreciation and Thankfulness

Introduction:

Gratitude is a important practice that cultivates a positive mindset, enhances well- being, and strengthens connections. It involves admitting and appreciating the good in our lives, both big and small. In this composition, we explore the transformative nature of gratefulness, examining its benefits, styles for cultivating gratefulness, and its profound impact on particular growth and connections. By embracing gratefulness and rehearsing appreciativeness, we can produce a fulfilling and joyous life.

Understanding Gratitude

Defining Gratitude
Gratitude is the practice of feting and admitting the virtuousness, kindness, and blessings in our lives. It involves

expressing appreciation for what we have, rather than fastening on what's lacking.

Gratitude as an station
Gratitude isn't simply an occasional feeling; it's a way of life. It's an station that can be cultivated and nurtured through conscious trouble and practice.

II. The Benefits of Gratitude

Emotional Well- being
Gratitude has a profound impact on our emotional well- being. It promotes positive feelings, reduces stress, anxiety, and depression, and increases overall life satisfaction and happiness.

Physical Health
Research has shown that gratefulness is linked to bettered physical health. rehearsing gratefulness is associated with better sleep quality, reduced blood pressure, enhanced vulnerable function, and dropped symptoms of illness.

III. Cultivating Gratitude

Keeping a Gratitude Journal

One effective system for cultivating gratefulness is to keep a gratefulness journal. This involves regularly writing down effects we're thankful for, reflecting on the positive aspects of our lives, and expressing gratefulness for the blessings we've entered.

Counting Blessings
Taking a moment each day to mentally or verbally count our blessings can help shift our focus from negativity to appreciation. By purposely admitting the good in our lives, we cultivate a sense of gratefulness.

rehearsing awareness
awareness involves being completely present in the moment and paying attention to our studies, passions, and gests . rehearsing aware gratefulness allows us to appreciate the present moment, savoring the simple mannas and beauty around us.

IV. The Power of Gratitude in connections

Strengthening Connections
Expressing gratefulness in connections strengthens the bond between

individualities. Showing appreciation for our favored bones
' presence, sweats, and support nurtures a sense of connection, love, and collective respect.

Cultivating Positivity
Gratitude fosters a positive atmosphere within connections. By admitting and expressing gratefulness for the positive rates and conduct of our mates, family, and musketeers, we produce an terrain of warmth and appreciation.

Gratitude and Personal Growth

Shifting Perspective
Gratitude helps shift our perspective from fastening on what's lacking to feting and appreciating what we have. This shift in mindset opens the door to particular growth, adaptability, and an cornucopia mindset.

Chancing Meaning and Purpose
Gratitude allows us to find meaning and purpose in our lives. By feting the value of our gests , connections, and openings, we gain a deeper sense of fulfillment and a lesser understanding of our life's purpose.

VI. Spreading Gratitude and Kindness

Paying It Forward
rehearsing gratefulness involves not only feting the good in our own lives but also extending kindness and gratefulness to others. Acts of kindness, arbitrary acts of liberality, and expressing gratefulness to others produce a positive ripple effect, spreading joy and inspiring gratefulness in others.

Creating a Culture of Gratitude
Cultivating a culture of gratefulness within our communities, workplaces, and families fosters an terrain of appreciation, collaboration, and well- being. By laboriously promoting gratefulness and feting the benefactions of others, we produce a harmonious and probative social fabric.

VII. prostrating Challenges and Finding Gratitude

Chancing Silver Linings
Gratitude can help us find tableware stuffings in grueling situations. By searching for the assignments and growth

openings within adversity, we can cultivate gratefulness indeed during delicate times.

Embracing Resilience
Gratitude strengthens our adaptability in the face of challenges. It provides us with a positive outlook, allowing us to navigate obstacles with lesser sanguinity, perseverance, and determination.

VIII. Living a Grateful Life

Integrating Gratitude into Daily Practices
To truly live a thankful life, it's essential to integrate gratefulness into our diurnal practices. Making gratefulness a habit involves incorporating gratefulness rituals, expressing appreciation, and being aware of the blessings in our lives.

Embracing an Cornucopia Mindset
Gratitude helps cultivate an cornucopia mindset, shifting our focus from failure to cornucopia. By appreciating what we've and feting the possibilities and openings around us, we open ourselves to a world of cornucopia and fulfillment.

Chapter 11: Weeding out Negativity: Overcoming Destructive Patterns

Introduction:

Negativity and destructive patterns can insinuate our lives, affecting our well-being, connections, and overall happiness. Whether it manifests as tone-mistrustfulness, poisonous actions, or negative study patterns, these destructive patterns can hamper particular growth and lead to a cycle of unhappiness. In this composition, we explore strategies for relating and prostrating negativity, empowering ourselves to break free from destructive patterns and cultivate a more positive and fulfilling life. By admitting negative patterns, rehearsing tone-mindfulness, seeking support, and embracing positive habits, we can weed out negativity and produce a life of positivity and growth.

relating Destructive Patterns

tone- Reflection
tone- reflection is pivotal in relating destructive patterns. Taking the time to examine our studies, feelings, and actions allows us to gain sapience into negative patterns that may be holding us back.

Feting Negative study Patterns
Negative study patterns, similar as tone- review, catastrophizing, or negative tone- talk, contribute to destructive patterns. relating and challenging these studies is essential for breaking free from negativity.

II. rehearsing tone- mindfulness

awareness
awareness involves being completely present and apprehensive of our studies, feelings, and sensations. By rehearsing awareness, we can observe negative patterns as they arise and make conscious choices to respond else.

Journaling
Journaling provides a space for tone- reflection and tone- expression. By

writing about our studies, passions, and gests , we can gain clarity, identify patterns, and develop strategies for prostrating negativity.

III. Challenging Negative Beliefs

Examining Core Beliefs
Core beliefs are deeply hardwired beliefs that shape our perception of ourselves, others, and the world. relating negative core beliefs and challenging their validity is a pivotal step in prostrating destructive patterns.

Reframing
Reframing involves purposely shifting our perspective on a situation. By looking for indispensable explanations or fastening on positive aspects, we can reframe negative gests and produce a further formative narrative.

IV. Cultivating Positive Habits

Gratitude Practice
Cultivating gratefulness through regular practice helps shift our focus from negativity to appreciation. By admitting the positive aspects of our lives, we

produce a more positive mindset and break free from negative patterns.

tone- Care Routine
Engaging in tone- care conditioning promotes physical and emotional well-being. Developing a tone- care routine that includes exercise, acceptable rest, healthy eating, and conditioning that bring joy and relaxation can help offset negativity.

Seeking Support

erecting a probative Network
girding ourselves with probative and positive individualities can help offset negativity. Having a network of trusted musketeers, family, or instructors who give stimulant, guidance, and emotional support is inestimable in prostrating destructive patterns.

Professional Help
In some cases, seeking professional help from therapists or trainers can give fresh guidance and support. These professionals are equipped with the tools and moxie to help individualities navigate and overcome destructive patterns.

VI. Setting Boundaries

relating poisonous connections
poisonous connections can immortalize
negativity and destructive patterns.
relating and distancing ourselves from
poisonous individualities is pivotal for
our well- being and particular growth.

Establishing particular Boundaries
Setting clear and healthy boundaries is
essential in precluding negativity from
insinuating our lives. Communicating our
requirements, saying no when necessary,
and guarding our emotional well- being
helps produce a positive and probative
terrain.

VII. Cultivating a Growth Mindset

Embracing literacy and Growth
espousing a growth mindset involves
believing in our capacity to learn, grow,
and change. Seeing challenges as
openings for growth and viewing lapses
as learning gests helps offset negativity
and fosters particular development.

Embracing Adaptability

Adaptability is the capability to bounce back from adversity. Cultivating adaptability involves developing managing strategies, seeking support when demanded, and maintaining a positive outlook indeed in the face of challenges.

VIII. Taking Responsibility for particular Growth

Accepting Responsibility
Overcoming destructive patterns requires taking responsibility for our studies, feelings, and actions. Admitting that we've the power to change and laboriously seeking growth empowers us to break free from negativity.

Committing to Personal Development
Making a commitment to particular development involves setting pretensions, seeking openings for literacy and tone- enhancement, and embracing challenges as openings for growth.

IX. thickness and continuity

enforcing Positive Change

Overcoming destructive patterns and cultivating positivity bear thickness and continuity. enforcing positive changes, similar as rehearsing gratefulness, challenging negative studies, and seeking support, on a regular base reinforces new patterns and helps break free from negativity.

Embracing the Journey
Overcoming destructive patterns is a trip that requires tolerance and tone-compassion. Embracing the ups and campo, celebrating progress, and learning from lapses contribute to long- term growth and metamorphosis.

Chapter 12: Nourishing Romance: Reigniting Passion and Desire

Introduction:

Romantic Connections are dynamic and ever- evolving, taking purposeful trouble to nurture and maintain passion and desire over time. While the original stages of love may be marked by excitement and intensity, it's natural for connections to go through phases where passion and desire may wane. still, with aware attention and deliberate conduct, couples can reignite the spark and cultivate a thriving, passionate connection. In this composition, we explore strategies for nutritional love, reigniting passion, and fostering a deeper sense of desire within a married relationship. By understanding the significance of emotional connection, embracing closeness, exploring new gests , and prioritizing tone- care, couples can embark on a trip of rejuvenating and sustaining a passionate and fulfilling relationship.

Understanding the Dynamics of Passion and Desire

The elaboration of Passion
Passion in a relationship frequently evolves over time. originally driven by passion and novelty, it transforms into a deeper emotional and intimate connection as the relationship progresses. Understanding the natural progression of passion is essential for cultivating long-term desire.

The part of Desire
Desire is the glamorous force that energies romantic connections. It encompasses physical magnet, emotional connection, and a sense of craving for one's mate. Nurturing desire requires a holistic approach that encompasses colorful aspects of the relationship.

II. Emotional Connection The Foundation of Passion

Cultivating Emotional closeness
Emotional closeness is the bedrock of a passionate relationship. Building trust, rehearsing active listening, expressing

vulnerability, and nurturing open communication are essential for fostering emotional connection and reigniting passion.

heightening Emotional Bond
Engaging in conditioning that foster emotional connection, similar as participating dreams and pretensions, ignoring about positive gests , and engaging in meaningful exchanges, helps strengthen the emotional bond between mates.

III. Embracing closeness The Pathway to Passion

Physical closeness
Physical closeness plays a vital part in nurturing desire. Engaging in tender touch, exploring new forms of physical connection, and prioritizing quality time for closeness can reignite passion and foster a deeper sense of desire.

voluptuous disquisition
Exploring hedonism beyond sexual closeness, similar as voluptuous massages, participated cataracts, or engaging in sensitive conditioning, can

enhance connection and reignite passion. voluptuous disquisition allows mates to reconnect and consolidate their physical and emotional bond.

IV. Rediscovering Shared Pleasures

rejuvenating Romance
Engaging in conditioning that bring back the passions of love and excitement can reignite passion. Planning surprise date nights, recreating memorable gests , or writing love letters can elicit the same passions endured during the early stages of the relationship.

audacious gests
participating new and stirring gests together can awaken passion and desire. Trying new conditioning, exploring new destinations, or engaging in participated pursuits or interests produce openings for cling and cultivating passion.

Communication and Vulnerability

Expressing solicitations and Fantasies
Open and honest communication about solicitations, fantasies, and preferences is essential for reigniting passion. Creating a

safe andnon-judgmental space where mates can partake their deepest solicitations fosters closeness and creates openings for exploring new confines of passion.

Emotional translucency
Being emotionally transparent with one another builds trust and deepens the connection. participating fears, precariousness, and vulnerabilities allows for lesser closeness and can reignite passion by creating a sense of emotional closeness.

VI. Prioritizing tone- Care

Individual Growth and Fulfillment
Prioritizing particular growth and tone- care enhances overall well- being and appreciatively impacts the relationship. Engaging in conditioning that promote tone- fulfillment, similar as pursuing pursuits, tone- reflection, and tone- enhancement, allows mates to bring a sense of sprightliness and passion into the relationship.

tone- Confidence and Body Positivity

Cultivating tone- confidence and embracing body positivity are crucial rudiments in fostering desire and reigniting passion. Embracing and celebrating one's own body helps produce a positive and confident energy that's seductive and charming to one's mate.

VII. Rediscovering Each Other

Date Nights and Quality Time

Setting away devoted time for date nights or quality time together allows mates to reconnect, memorize, and consolidate their emotional and physical bond. Creating a regular ritual of spending purposeful time together strengthens the foundation of passion and desire.

Rediscovering Interests and pursuits

Encouraging each other to pursue individual interests and pursuits helps mates maintain a sense of individuality and brings new gests and stories to partake within the relationship. This fosters a sense of excitement and newness, reigniting passion and desire.

VIII. Managing Relationship Challenges

Addressing Conflict
Effectively addressing and resolving
conflicts is pivotal for maintaining a
passionate relationship. Cultivating
healthy communication chops,
laboriously harkening, and chancing
formative results contribute to a more
harmonious and passionate connection.

Seeking Professional Help
In cases where relationship challenges
persist, seeking the guidance of a couples
therapist can give precious support.
Professional intervention offers a safe
space for exploring underpinning issues
and developing strategies to reignite
passion and desire.

IX. Embracing Inflexibility and
elaboration

Embracing Change and Growth
Feting that connections evolve over time
and embracing change is vital for
sustaining passion and desire. Being open
to growth, both collectively and as a
couple, allows for the discovery of new
aspects of the relationship and the
nonstop development of desire.

Cultivating Gratitude
Expressing gratefulness for one another and the relationship fosters a positive and appreciative mindset. Gratitude reminds mates of the value they bring to each other's lives and nurtures a sense of passion and desire.

Chapter 13: Embracing Growth: Supporting Each Other's Personal Development

Introduction:

A strong and fulfilling relationship is one that not only nurtures love and fellowship but also supports the particular growth and development of each existent. When mates laboriously embrace particular growth and encourage each other's trip of tone- enhancement, the relationship thrives and evolves. In this composition, we claw into the significance of embracing growth within a relationship, exploring strategies for supporting each other's particular development. From fostering open communication and setting participated pretensions to furnishing emotional support and creating a nurturing terrain, we uncover the transformative power of supporting one another's particular growth and cultivating a relationship that's innovated on collective growth, understanding, and stimulant.

Understanding Personal Development in a Relationship

Defining Personal Development
Personal development refers to the lifelong process of tone- enhancement, tone- discovery, and growth. It encompasses colorful aspects, including emotional, intellectual, physical, and spiritual growth.

Embracing Individuality within a Relationship
Supporting particular development in a relationship involves feting and recognizing each mate's unique identity, heartstrings, and pretensions. It requires embracing individuality while maintaining a strong sense of togetherness.

II. Fostering Open Communication

Active harkening
Active listening is a abecedarian aspect of supporting particular development. furnishing concentrated attention,

empathetically harkening, and encouraging open dialogue creates a safe space for mates to partake their bournes , fears, and growth gests .

participating pretensions and Dreams Encouraging mates to openly communicate their pretensions, dreams, and bournes allows for a participated vision of particular growth. participating these bournes fosters collective understanding, support, and responsibility.

III. furnishing Emotional Support

Empathy and Understanding furnishing emotional support involves empathizing with each other's challenges, triumphs, and feelings. Demonstrating understanding and validating each other's gests produce a nurturing terrain for particular growth.

Celebrating Achievements Celebrating each other's mileposts and achievements is pivotal for fostering particular growth. Admitting and celebrating the progress made in individual pretensions strengthens the sense of accomplishment and motivates farther growth.

IV. Creating a Nurturing Environment

collective Respect
A nurturing terrain is erected on collective respect. Valuing each other's studies, beliefs, and boundaries fosters a sense of safety and encourages particular disquisition and growth.

Encouraging Autonomy
Supporting particular development involves empowering mates to make independent choices and opinions. Encouraging autonomy fosters tone-confidence and a sense of commission.

Building on Strengths

relating Strengths
Supporting particular development involves feting and encouraging each other's strengths. relating and nurturing these strengths contribute to a sense of purpose, tone- worth, and fulfillment.

uniting and Learning Together

mates can support each other's growth by collaboratively learning and participating knowledge. Engaging in common conditioning, similar as attending shops or taking courses together, promotes growth and strengthens the relationship.

VI. Challenging and Inspiring Each Other

Encouraging threat- Taking
Supporting particular development frequently requires taking pitfalls. Encouraging each other to step outside of comfort zones and pursue new challenges promotes particular growth and fosters adaptability.

furnishing Formative Feedback
Offering formative feedback is essential for growth. furnishing honest feedback with kindness and respect allows mates to learn from their gests and make advancements.

VII. Balancing Individual and Relationship Needs

Setting Boundaries
Supporting particular development involves setting healthy boundaries that

admire each mate's need for particular space, time, and growth. Chancing a balance between individual and participated conditioning promotes a sense of autonomy within the relationship.

participating liabilities
Balancing individual growth with participated liabilities strengthens the relationship. uniting on ménage tasks, fiscal operation, and decision- making fosters an terrain where particular growth can flourish.

VIII. Encouraging tone- Care

Prioritizing Well- being
Supporting particular development requires prioritizing tone- care. Encouraging each other to engage in conditioning that promote physical, emotional, and internal well- being cultivates a foundation for particular growth.

Promoting Balance
Encouraging mates to find a healthy balance between work, connections, and particular interests is essential for

sustaining particular growth. Balancing colorful aspects of life prevents collapse and nurtures well- rounded growth.

IX. prostrating Challenges and Supporting Adaptability

Navigating lapses
Supporting particular development involves helping each other navigate lapses and challenges. Offering emotional support, brainstorming results, and furnishing stimulant during delicate times foster adaptability and growth.

Seeking Professional Help
In grueling situations, seeking the guidance of professionals, similar as therapists or trainers, can give precious support. Professional intervention offers fresh tools and perceptivity to navigate obstacles and promote particular development.

Celebrating Growth and Reflection

Reflecting on particular Growth
Taking time to reflect on particular growth allows mates to celebrate progress, identify areas for enhancement,

and set new pretensions. Reflective practices, similar as journaling or regular check- sways, grease ongoing particular development.

Celebrating mileposts
Celebrating particular growth mileposts and achievements is essential for fostering a probative and growth- acquainted relationship. Marking these mileposts together strengthens the bond and encourages continued growth.

Chapter 14: Seasons of Love: Adapting to Change and Embracing Transitions

Introduction:

Love is a trip that takes us through different seasons, marked by change, growth, and transitions. From the exhilarating days of new love to the challenges and growth that come with time, connections go through colorful seasons. conforming to these changes and embracing transitions is essential for maintaining a healthy and thriving cooperation. In this composition, we explore the conception of seasons of love, probing into the significance of conforming to change, navigating transitions, and fostering adaptability within connections. By understanding the nature of transitions, embracing communication and inflexibility, fostering emotional adaptability, and prioritizing growth together, couples can navigate the seasons of love and produce a relationship that thrives in every stage.

Understanding the Seasons of Love

The Cycle of Change
connections witness different seasons, much like the changing seasons in nature. These seasons encompass the highs and lows, growth and challenges, and the ever- evolving nature of love.

Feting Transitions
Transitions do when connections move from one season to another. These transitions can be marked by mileposts, life events, or shifts in dynamics and bear adaption and adaptation.

II. Embracing Communication and Inflexibility

Open and Honest Communication
Effective communication is vital in navigating the seasons of love. Regularly expressing studies, passions, and needs allows couples to understand and support each other through transitions.

Inflexibility and Rigidity

Embracing inflexibility is crucial when facing change and transitions. Being open to new possibilities, conforming prospects, and embracing change together enables couples to navigate the shifting seasons of love.

III. Navigating Major Life Events

Birth of Children
The appearance of children is a significant life event that brings both joy and challenges. conforming to parenting involves communication, participated liabilities, and chancing a balance between individual and maternal places.

Career Changes
Career changes can impact connections by introducing new routines, challenges, and shifts in dynamics. Open communication and support during these transitions foster understanding and growth.

Relocation
shifting to a new megacity or country can bring about significant changes in a relationship. erecting a new support network, conforming to a new terrain,

and navigating artistic adaptations bear open communication, tolerance, and support.

IV. Fostering Emotional Adaptability

structure Emotional Adaptability
Emotional adaptability is pivotal in navigating the seasons of love. structure adaptability involves developing managing mechanisms, managing stress, and seeking support during grueling times.

Cultivating Empathy and Compassion
Embracing empathy and compassion allows mates to support each other through the ups and campo of different seasons. By understanding each other's feelings and perspectives, couples foster emotional adaptability.

Prioritizing Growth and Self- Care

particular Growth
Prioritizing particular growth within a relationship is essential for navigating seasons of love. Setting individual pretensions, pursuing pursuits and interests, and seeking particular

fulfillment contribute to the overall well-being of the relationship.

tone- Care Practices
Engaging in tone- care practices is vital for maintaining a healthy and balanced relationship. Prioritizing physical, emotional, and internal well- being allows couples to face transitions with adaptability and rigidity.

VI. Cultivating closeness and Connection

Quality Time
Making purposeful time for each other strengthens the bond and fosters closeness. Setting away regular quality time helps couples navigate transitions by nurturing emotional connection and support.

closeness and Physical Affection
Maintaining closeness and physical affection is pivotal in all seasons of love. Being attentive to each other's requirements and solicitations, and openly communicating about closeness fosters a deeper sense of connection and closeness.

VII. Seeking Support and Professional Guidance

Seeking Support from musketeers and Family
musketeers and family can give a precious support system during different seasons of love. Seeking advice, participating gests , and leaning on loved bones
help couples navigate transitions with a sense of community.

Professional Guidance
In grueling times or during significant transitions, seeking professional guidance from therapists or relationship counselors can offer tools, perceptivity, and strategies for navigating the seasons of love.

VIII. Embracing the Power of concession and Collaboration

concession in Decision- Making
Successful navigation of the seasons of love frequently involves concession. Being willing to make negotiations and chancing palm- palm results contribute to a harmonious and adaptable relationship.

cooperative Problem- working
Embracing cooperative problem- working allows couples to attack challenges together. By approaching issues as a platoon, couples can navigate transitions with collective support and understanding.

IX. Appreciating the Journey

Gratitude and Reflection
rehearsing gratefulness and reflecting on the trip of love fosters appreciation for the growth and gests participated. Taking time to celebrate mileposts and express gratefulness strengthens the bond and deepens the connection.

Embracing the Present Moment
Embracing the present moment allows couples to completely witness and savor each season of love. By being present, couples can cultivate a deeper sense of connection and joy in the trip.

Embracing Change and Growth Together

Supporting Individual pretensions

Supporting each other's existent pretensions and dreams promotes particular growth within the relationship. Encouraging and empowering one another creates a probative terrain for growth and fulfillment.

Shared Growth
Nurturing participated pretensions and bournes allows couples to grow together. uniting on participated systems, setting common pretensions, and pursuing collective interests foster a sense of concinnity and nonstop growth.

Chapter 15: The Evergreen Bond: Sustaining Love and Commitment Throughout a Lifetime

Introduction:

Love is a trip that evolves and matures over time, and sustaining a deep and fulfilling bond throughout a continuance requires fidelity, trouble, and a commitment to growth. erecting an evergreen bond involves nurturing love, fostering emotional connection, and continuously investing in the relationship. In this composition, we explore strategies for sustaining love and commitment throughout a continuance. From cultivating open communication and trust to embracing participated values and creating rituals of connection, we uncover the keys to erecting an evergreen bond that withstands the test of time.

Cultivating Emotional Connection

Prioritizing Emotional closeness
Emotional closeness is the foundation of a lasting bond. Prioritizing deep and meaningful exchanges, participating vulnerabilities, and laboriously harkening to one another fosters emotional connection and strengthens the relationship.

rehearsing Empathy and Understanding
Cultivating empathy and understanding allows mates to see effects from each other's perspectives. By laboriously trying to understand each other's passions and gests , couples consolidate their emotional connection and make a sense of collective support.

II. Embracing Open Communication

Honesty and Authenticity
Open and honest communication is pivotal in sustaining love throughout a continuance. Creating a safe space for vulnerability and expressing studies, passions, and needs without judgment fosters trust and understanding.

Active harkening

Active listening involves giving concentrated attention, validating each other's feelings, and seeking to understand before responding. By rehearsing active listening, couples can strengthen their communication and consolidate their connection.

III. Nurturing Trust and Security

thickness and trustability
thickness and trustability are vital for erecting trust in a relationship. recognizing commitments, being reliable, and following through on pledges creates a sense of security and fosters trust and commitment.

remission and Acceptance
Nurturing a forgiving and accepting mindset allows couples to overcome challenges and conflicts. Embracing remission and accepting each other's defects creates a safe terrain for growth and sustains love throughout a continuance.

IV. Embracing Shared Values and pretensions

Shared Values
Shared values produce a strong foundation for a lasting bond. Aligning on abecedarian beliefs and principles allows couples to navigate life's challenges and make opinions together grounded on a participated vision.

Setting Common pretensions
Setting common pretensions and bournes fosters a sense of concinnity and participated purpose. Working towards participated pretensions strengthens the bond and keeps the relationship dynamic and fulfilling.

Creating Rituals of Connection

Quality Time
sculpturing out devoted quality time for each other is essential for sustaining love. Whether through regular date nights, participated conditioning, or simply spending time together, rituals of connection consolidate emotional bonds and produce lasting recollections.

Expressing Affection
Expressing affection through physical touch, words of protestation, or acts of

kindness reinforces the love and commitment between mates. Regular displays of affection nurture the emotional connection and sustain love over time.

VI. Embracing Growth and Rigidity

Embracing Individual Growth
Supporting each other's particular growth and allowing space for individual hobbies contributes to the life of love.
Encouraging particular development and celebrating achievements fosters a sense of fulfillment within the relationship.

conforming to Life Changes
Life is full of transitions and changes, and conforming together is pivotal for sustaining love. Whether it's career changes, parenting, or health challenges, facing life's ups and campo as a platoon strengthens the bond and reinforces commitment.

VII. rehearsing Gratitude and Appreciation

Expressing Gratitude

Regularly expressing gratefulness for one another and the relationship cultivates a positive and appreciative mindset. Admitting and celebrating each other's benefactions and expressing gratefulness for the love and support entered nourishes the bond.

Appreciating the Little effects
Paying attention to and appreciating the small gestures, kindnesses, and moments of joy in diurnal life enriches the relationship. Feting and valuing the small moments of connection sustains love throughout a continuance.

VIII. Seeking Support and Seeking Help

Seeking Support from Loved Bones
structure a support network of family and musketeers who encourage and celebrate the relationship enhances its life. participating gests , seeking advice, and chancing alleviation from loved bones strengthen the bond.

Seeking Professional Help
In times of significant challenges or when the relationship faces obstacles, seeking the guidance of a professional therapist or

counselor can give precious tools and perceptivity to navigate difficulties and sustain love.

IX. Prioritizing tone- Care and Well- being

Individual tone- Care
Prioritizing individual tone- care and well- being is pivotal for sustaining love in the long run. Nurturing physical, emotional, and internal well- being allows mates to show up completely in the relationship and contribute to its growth.

Shared Self- Care
Engaging in participated tone- care conditioning promotes connection and enhances the bond. Encouraging each other to prioritize tone- care and engaging in conditioning together that promote well- being strengthens the relationship.

Celebrating mileposts and Cherishing Memories

Celebrating mileposts
Marking mileposts and celebrating achievements together reinforces the bond and creates lasting recollections.

Celebrating anniversaries, accomplishments, and participated gests brings joy and a sense of accomplishment to the relationship.

Cherishing Memories
Taking time to memorize and cherish recollections fosters a sense of gratefulness and love. Reflecting on the trip traveled together and celebrating the growth and mileposts strengthens the bond and sustains love throughout a continuance.

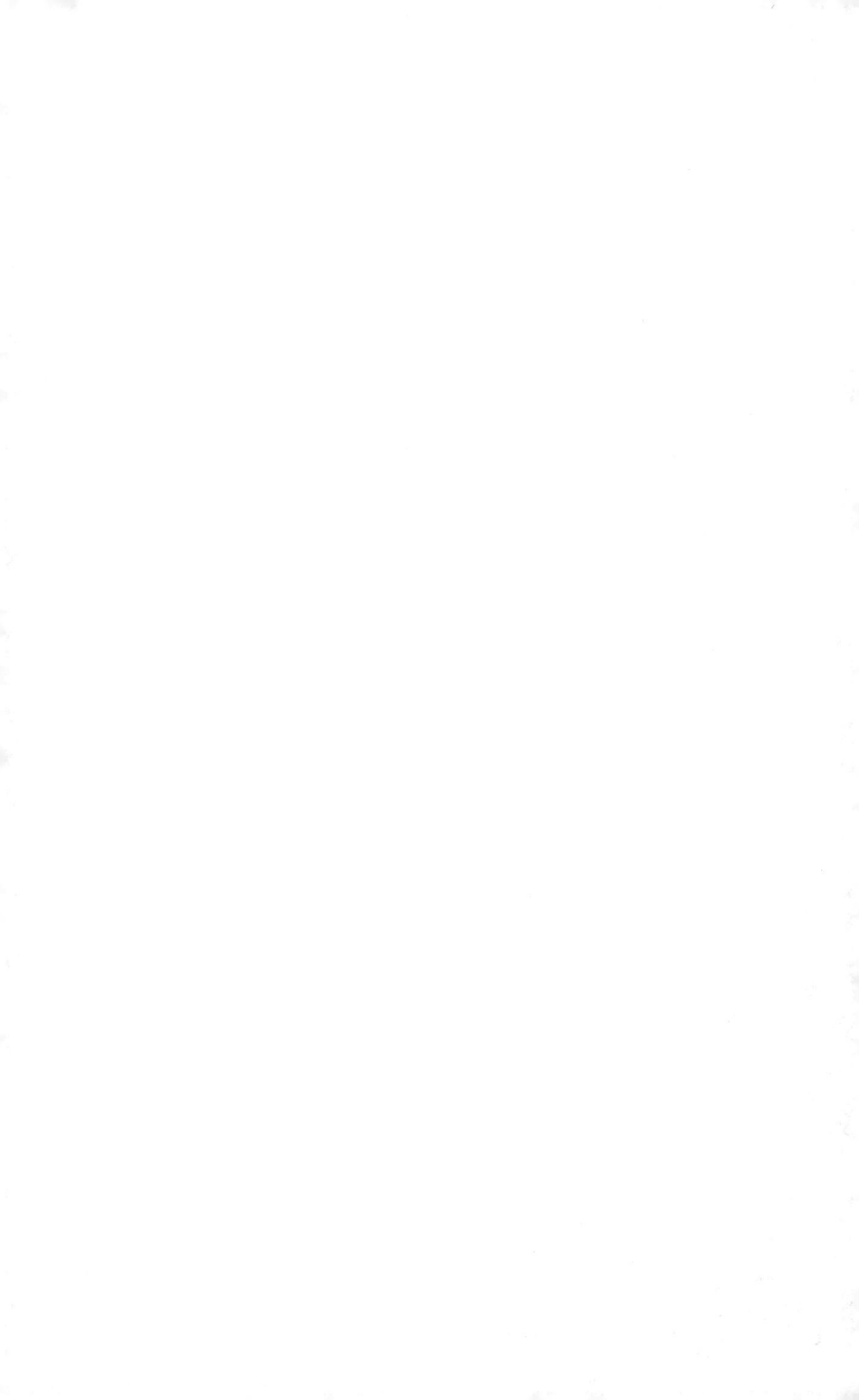

www.ingramcontent.com/pod-product-compliance
Lightning Source LLC
Chambersburg PA
CBHW062348290526
45794CB00005B/2140